DEALING WITH STRESS

The 'Mind, Body, Spirit' Way

A Simple Guide to Stress

by

Dr. Rebecca Williams

www.williamsstressmanagement.co.uk

3rd Edition

INTRODUCTION

At a time when individuals, couples and families are facing a multitude of pressures and worries, stress is becoming a real problem for many people.

Stress is a word that is used a lot but what does it actually mean? It can be defined as a mental, physical and/or emotional response to a situation and/or event/s which results in tension in the mind, body and/or spirit. A stressor, therefore, is essentially anything that causes stress. A stressor makes someone feel stressed by making them feel anxious or worried, or under too much pressure, or both. Some people struggle when they are under pressure, while others are motivated and energised by it. However, even those individuals who thrive will eventually reach a point beyond which the pressure becomes too much and becomes stressful.

There are many factors which may contribute to a person feeling stressed. They include the lack of control they may feel over their situation, having too much to do and no time to recharge, painful things which have happened in the past and fears regarding the future.

When a person is stressed, it affects their mind (thoughts and thinking habits), their body (resulting in a variety of physical symptoms) and their spirit (that part of us tied up with our emotions and how we feel). All are linked and overlap.

The aim of this book is to help you identify the following:-

Stressors in your life.

The impact stress can have on your health.

What you can do to help yourself lessen the negative impact of stress on your life.

I hope that this book will help you become more self-aware so that you can make the necessary changes in yourself and, wherever possible, in your situation, to make life less stressful.

THE FIGHT OR FLIGHT RESPONSE

The Fight or Flight response (also known as the Acute Stress Response) is an extremely important evolutionary adaptation which allows people to respond to life threatening situations with increased strength and speed; also with heightened senses (such as vision and hearing) and increased alertness. It is a highly complex response which I will try to keep simple for the purposes of this book.

When the brain receives messages from the outside world, via the senses, it processes them. If the situation is deemed dangerous, there are rapid changes enabling a dramatic response. These changes occur in the brain and the body, activating systems which are helpful but, at the same time, suppressing systems which are not needed in this dynamic situation. Once the threat is over, the body and brain revert to their natural resting states.

This incredible Acute Stress Response frequently saves lives. However, where someone is experiencing chronic stress/anxiety, many of these same changes within the body and brain are triggered and are then maintained for long periods of time. It is no surprise, therefore, that chronic stress and anxiety can impact on physical and mental health.

CAN STRESSORS BE CHANGED OR AVOIDED?

The quote below is from the Serenity Prayer, originally written by Reinhold Niebuhr (1892-1971). It might help you to read it and think about what it means and how it relates to your situation:

'Grant me the serenity to accept the things I cannot change, the courage to change the things I can and the wisdom to know the difference'.

List the stressors in your life in the space below.

If there are stressors which you are in a position to change, focus your energies on doing what you need to do, or can do, to create change. Examples might include looking for a new job, reducing your working hours, getting help to care for a loved one, seeking financial advice, reporting bullying at work, making time to reconnect with your partner, making up after a disagreement or letting go of some commitments to free up time.

Identify those stressors on your list which you are in a position to do something about and think about how you can change the situation. Make a plan in the space below.

If, however, the stressor/s cannot be changed, you need to focus your energies on changing your response to the source of your stress. By finding ways to build yourself up you will become stronger in facing your situation. The rest of this book is designed to help you do this.

HOW DOES STRESS AFFECT YOUR MIND, BODY AND SPIRIT?

YOUR MIND

When people are stressed, they are often distracted, they find it difficult to concentrate and are prone to memory lapses. However, often the mind goes into overdrive and can become dominated by anxious and negative thoughts which can feel overwhelming at times.
(It is worth noting that a general tendency towards anxious and negative thoughts can predispose people to stress.)

Do you have a tendency towards any of the following?

A glass half empty approach, tending to focus on the negatives of a situation.

Worrying about what other people think about you.

Lacking confidence in your abilities and a tendency to focus on your perceived weaknesses.

To catastrophise. (Fixating on worst case scenarios)

To minimise. (Not taking something seriously)

To blame yourself for things, even though they are not your fault.

To seek perfection and to feel a failure if you haven't done things perfectly.

To make assumptions about your day, based on how you feel. e.g. I feel fed up so today won't go well.

To disqualify the positives. e.g. They're only saying that because they feel sorry for me.

Overgeneralising. e.g. No-one likes me.

Mind-reading: Assuming you know what someone is thinking. e.g. They think I talk too much.

Making assumptions which are not based on fact. e.g. They're going to fire me.

These are unhealthy thinking patterns that can have a significant impact on how you live your life and, ultimately, on your health.

Use the space below to write down thoughts that have been in the forefront of your mind recently.

YOUR BODY

Stress can affect many parts of your body in a negative way. Examples include:-

Headaches: Tension headaches (a feeling of pressure at the front of the head and over the top, like a vice) and migraines (classically a thumping headache often associated with intolerance of light).

Viral and bacterial infections: These include cold-sores, shingles, coughs/colds, chest infections.

Skin: Flare ups in psoriasis and eczema, non-specific rashes.

Bowels: Bowel symptoms are commonly caused by anxiety/stress. Irritable Bowel Syndrome (IBS) is characterised by bloating, constipation, diarrhoea and abdominal cramps. Other symptoms include heartburn and indigestion.

Heart/breathing: Racing heart-rate, thumping heart beats, shallow/rapid breathing, chest pains (panic attacks are classically associated with anxiety/stress).

Back/Neck: Muscle tension/spasm.

Blood Pressure: long periods of stress can result in an increase in blood pressure without giving rise to any symptoms. However, left untreated, high blood pressure can cause significant health problems.

Other: Fatigue, loss of appetite.

If you have been aware of any of these symptoms, list them in the space below. Do you need a blood pressure check?

OUR SPIRIT

The effect of stress on the spirit gives rise to the following feelings: low, impatient, irritable, tearful, as if 'nothing left to give', as if 'running on empty'.

Have you been feeling any of these?

UNHEALTHY COPING BEHAVIOURS

Coping behaviours are the things that people do to help them cope with challenging times and to feel better. Most of this book is about healthy ways of coping with life and, particularly, with stress. However, I must touch on unhealthy coping behaviours because these have the potential to cause harm to health.

Caffeine: Caffeinated drinks (including green tea!) are commonly used to help people get through the day, especially if they are not sleeping well. However, caffeine is a stimulant so can increase the risk of palpitations and panic attacks. It also makes people pass more urine so increases the risk of dehydration and urine infections.

Sugary and fatty snacks/meals: These foods are highly calorific so if eaten in large quantities will increase the risk of weight gain and the medical conditions associated with being overweight or obese. These conditions include diabetes and the lesser well known NAFLD (non-alcoholic fatty liver disease) in which abdominal fat is deposited in the liver and can cause damage to the liver very similar to that caused by alcohol.

Alcohol: People use alcohol for a variety of reasons, when life is tough. It is used to help people to relax, to calm anxieties in particular situations, as a treat after a hard day and to help sleep. However, alcohol can cause significant damage to the liver and is highly calorific, contributing to weight issues. It is also potentially addictive and the power of addiction can destroy lives at many levels.

Medication for anxiety/sleep: Many patients ask their GP for tablets to help them with anxiety or to help them sleep. Some people obtain these tablets online. Whilst there are tablets effective at treating these issues, they are highly addictive. They should only be taken in small quantities for short term or emergency use. It is far better to follow the advice in this book for managing anxiety and poor sleep.

Other unhealthy coping behaviours: Many people find ways to 'escape' or 'feel good' as a means of coping with stress. Shopping, sex, drugs and gambling are common and can quickly become addictive. As with all addictions, it doesn't take long for these habits to generate a significant negative impact on someone's life.

List any unhealthy coping behaviours you have, in the space below. Do any of them need attention?

Having read the first part of this book, I hope you are now able to identify the stressors in your life and to recognise how stress affects your mental, physical and emotional health. When it comes to improving your health, it is important to consider the big picture and not simply to focus on your particular symptom/s. Remember, the effects of stress interact. For example, anxious and negative thinking patterns can worsen physical symptoms such as muscle tension, panic symptoms and bowel symptoms. Physical symptoms can impact on mental and emotional health. To lessen the impact of stress on your health, I would encourage you to use this book to help you nurture your mental, physical and emotional health as a whole and not simply to focus on treating symptoms.

LOOKING AFTER YOUR MIND

The way people think affects the way they feel and the way they live. It is important to protect minds and to control negative thinking patterns. Antidepressants and anti-anxiety medication can also have a role to play in helping but need to be used alongside the other tools I am describing.

Below is some advice on how to tackle negative and anxious thoughts:

Try to become more aware of your thoughts in different situations. Remember the list earlier in the book. Are you aware of any of these thoughts in yourself? Are you mulling on negatives? Do you just keep wishing the situation was different or would go away? Are you worrying about what others think of you? Are you lacking confidence in yourself and putting yourself down?

If you recognise any of the these thinking patterns, it is important that you take action because, left unchecked, negative and anxious thinking patterns can dominate your mind and have a profoundly negative impact on your mental and physical health. Here are some tips on things you can do.

Protect your mind:-

Minimise the amount of time you spend reading news stories or social media posts that make you feel sad or anxious. Focus on good news and uplifting or interesting stories.

Ensure you are reading information from trusted and reliable sources.

When you communicate with friends and family, try to discuss positive and encouraging things. Offload if you need to but don't spend all your time talking about things that make you feel sad or anxious.

Control your anxious and negative thoughts:-

Challenge them: Try to look at your situation from a different perspective and find other explanations. For example, don't assume someone doesn't like you or that you've done something wrong. Challenging negative or anxious thoughts is the basis for CBT (Cognitive Behavioural Therapy). It is a technique that is now widely available to help people and there are many books and on-line resources that can facilitate the management of anxiety and stress using this technique.

Distraction: Find something to distract you from your negative and anxious thoughts. For example, a sudoku, a crossword, a game on your phone, looking at photos, talking to someone.

Catchphrase: Find a phrase that helps you break a negative thinking cycle. For example, 'Let it go', 'I'm not going there'.

Happy Place: Find a real or imagined happy place in your mind that you can go to when you're feeling stressed. Picture it and imagine you are there.

Encourage positive thinking:-

'Post it' notes: Put them around your house and whenever you see one say something positive to yourself about yourself or something you are grateful for. You can modify this idea to suit you. For example, say something positive whenever you use your phone or go through a door. If you are struggling to think of positive things to say about yourself, ask your friends and family what they love about you and write down what they say. If will be

a useful list of affirmations to build you up when you're finding things hard.

Gratitude journal: Keep a notebook where you write down the things you are grateful for. Some people find this useful to do routinely every night before they go to sleep, noting 3 to 5 things daily.

Positive quotes: If you google 'positive quotes' you will find a whole load of them. Jot down the ones you like in a notebook and keep it with you to look at when you are struggling.

Other tools:-

Meditation and Mindfulness techniques can be very helpful in calming the mind. You can look on-line for ideas or attend a class. They aim to help you focus on the moment, free of the clutter of the past and fears for the future. (There is a simple mindfulness exercise at the end of the book).

By taking action, you can train your thinking patterns to become less negative and anxious, thereby creating a calmer and more positive mind. Change won't happen overnight so you will need to be willing to persevere, but it will be worth it in the long run.

LOOKING AFTER YOUR BODY

General advice:-

Nutrition: It is important to ensure that your body is being nourished and hydrated. Good habits to get into include:-

Eating regular meals (try not to miss meals, avoid large meals late at night).
Eating balanced meals with plenty of fruit and veg.
Taking a break from work at mealtimes.
Minimising snacking on sugary and fatty foods.
Minimising alcohol and caffeine intake.
Drinking plenty of clear fluids (water, juice) to keep your body well hydrated.

Some people may want to attend a health food shop or speak to a nutritionist to discuss specific dietary issues further.

Relaxation: Finding time to relax is very important in dealing with stress. This may involve listening to music, watching TV, reading or just sitting and doing nothing. Whatever works best for you. Yoga can be helpful, as can acupuncture, massage and a variety of other complementary therapies, if financially feasible.

Physical Exercise: For a lot of people, physical exercise is a great stress reliever. There are many options available including running, walking, cycling, swimming, exercise classes, zumba classes and the gym. Some people prefer to exercise on their own, others find a class with other people more therapeutic. Find the form of exercise which works for you.

Sleep Advice: Stress often leads to lack of sleep, which makes everything worse. Some simple advice may help:-

1. Consider earplugs, blackout blinds and eye masks if you are sensitive to sound and light.

2. Consider sleeping in a different bed from your spouse/partner for a while if their presence affects your sleep.

3. Try to give yourself a wind-down period before going to bed aimed at resting your mind and body: have a break after any work you are doing, before going to bed; avoid watching anything too exciting or scary on TV; avoid caffeine after about 4pm; consider a long soak in the bath or listening to gentle music.

4. As you get into bed try not to worry about not sleeping as this will make it harder for you to get to sleep. Tell yourself it doesn't matter if you don't sleep well, even if you don't believe it, as it will keep you calm and more relaxed.

5. Keep a notepad and pen by your bed and if you suddenly think of something you need to remember for the next day, jot it down on your pad.

6. A glass of water by your bed can be useful, but only take sips.

7. Consider breathing exercises to calm your body. (See section on breathing exercises at the end of the book)

8. Consider sleep exercises designed to calm the mind. (An example has been given at the end of this book).

Specific advice for particular stress related conditions:-

Breathing: When people are stressed, they tend to breathe with shallow breaths which can result in breathlessness, light-headedness, palpitations and chest wall pains as well as full-blown panic attacks and tension in their body. Breathing exercises are really important in helping to relax mind and body and can play an important role in reducing the impact of stress. I have listed a selection of breathing exercises at the end of this book. You can get more information about these techniques on the internet or by joining a yoga class.

Panic attacks: For people struggling with panic attacks, breathing exercises are fundamental in reducing the frequency and severity of attacks. I recommend you use the techniques which work for you on a regular basis. In addition, I would suggest you carry a paper bag with you at all times and when you feel an actual panic attack coming on, breathe in and out of the paper bag and it will calm you.

Irritable Bowel Syndrome/bowel symptoms: I would suggest avoiding caffeine and spicy foods as they can exacerbate bowel symptoms. Be aware of any other trigger foods. If your symptoms are related to anxiety, use some of the techniques I have already described in this book to help you calm your mind and this, in turn, may improve your bowel symptoms.

Skin: If skin is flaring up, dietary factors can sometimes be an issue. You may want to discuss this matter at a health food shop or pay to speak to a nutritionist. Otherwise, ensure good moisturising and fluid intake.

Back/neck: When the back and neck are tense there are a number of physical treatments that can help. It might be worthwhile to pay for a good massage, acupuncture or other complementary therapies which can help with muscle tension. Simple measures such as heat and gentle stretches can also help (e.g. lie on back and bend knees to chest; gentle neck stretches). Remember that breathing techniques which help relax the body can also help reduce tension in the back and neck.

Migraine: In some people, migraines are a classic reaction to stress. It is important to find time for relaxation and to avoid trigger foods.

Tension headaches: These often result from stress and anxiety. It is important to tackle the negative thinking patterns as well as finding time to relax and to enjoy life.

RESTORING YOUR SPIRIT

This section is a very individual one. It is about you, as an individual, recognising what gives you joy and what helps you feel re-charged. The message is essentially, 'be kind to yourself, pamper yourself, and it is ok to put yourself first'. If you are 'running on empty,' you have nothing to give to anyone else. Sometimes you just have to put yourself first in order to recharge your batteries for the challenges you are facing and to renew your energy to give to others.

What makes you feel good inside? What do you enjoy?

Examples might include: walks, nature, a coffee shop with a friend or a book; buying yourself a bunch of flowers, listening to music, taking the dog for a walk, going fishing/playing golf, taking photos, going shopping for enjoyment, going for a run, spending quality time with the important people in your life.

Jot down the things you enjoy in the space below and find time to indulge in these things!

Focus on **enjoying the moment** and shutting off any worrying or negative thoughts. Focus on the little things in life that can bring enjoyment such as smiles on faces, colourful flowers and birdsong.

Helping others is also a good way feel uplifted as well as distracting you from your own stresses.

Some people have a Faith and may find services, prayer and talking to their Faith leader helpful.

(If you continue to struggle with your mental and/or physical health, despite your best efforts, it would be advisable to see your GP for further assessment).

GENERAL ADVICE

Spend time with people who make you feel good about yourself: Not with people who want something from you, who criticise you or who will drag you down.

Let others help: It is amazing how difficult many people find it to admit to themselves, and to others, when they are struggling. It is so important to find the courage to do so. Let close friends and family know how you are feeling and let them help. Ask for their help if you need to.

Learning to say 'no': Sometimes you just have to say 'no'. If you are running on empty and have nothing to give, it is not selfish to say 'no'. It is simply a realisation that if you don't take time to restore yourself, you'll have nothing left to give anyone. Try to find the courage to say 'no' when asked to do something and even let a previous commitment/s go. Hopefully, if you let people know that you are struggling and need time to recharge, they will understand.

Talking: Although it might seem scary, it can be a great help to talk about how you feel to someone you trust. This person may be a family member or a close friend. Other sources of listening support include your GP and counsellors, including relationship counsellors and bereavement counsellors.

FINALLY

Although this book is essentially designed to help in dealing with stress, I hope it will help you gain a greater understanding of yourself as a person.

I recommend making time on a regular basis, to 'check-in' on yourself. For example, an hour's slot in your diary once a month. Here is a 'check-in' framework you can use, should you want to:-

Identify your stressors and write them down.

Use the Serenity Prayer to remind you to focus your attention on the stressors which you are in a position to change and make a plan.

Reflect on any unhealthy coping behaviours and whether you need to moderate them.

Reflect on your thinking patterns and whether you have negative or anxious thinking patterns which need attention.

Reflect on your physical health and whether you are following the guidance given in this book. Are there things you need to change?

Reflect on your emotional health. Are you making time to do things that you enjoy and which help to recharge you?

This book should help you make the changes you need to make. Also, you might want to consider finding out more about things that could be of benefit e.g. CBT, mindfulness, yoga, physical exercise options.

By finding the time to 'check-in' on yourself you will gain a greater understanding of who you are and what you need to do to minimise the negative impact of stress on your life. By making the time to keep your batteries charged and having the courage to ask for help when you need it, you will be better equipped to deal with stressors as they arise in your life and are less likely to reach a crisis point. I hope this book will help you get into new habits so that you can look after your mind, your body and your spirit and can face the challenges ahead with renewed strength.

SLEEP EXERCISE

This exercise is designed to help calm your mind and bring your thoughts under control. It requires considerable concentration.

With your eyes closed and without speaking out loud, say the following to yourself, all the time focussing your thoughts on what you are saying and picturing what you are saying:

I am imagining the space between my eyes (repeat 3 times)

I am imagining the space between my ears (repeat 3 times)

I am imagining the space between my shoulders (repeat 3 times)

I am imagining the space between my elbows (repeat 3 times)

I am imagining the space between my hands (repeat 3 times)

I am imagining the space between my hips (repeat 3 times)

I am imagining the space between my knees (repeat 3 times)

I am imagining the space between my feet (repeat 3 times)

As you are doing this, other thoughts may try to interrupt you so you will have to be very strong minded and keep focussing on the exercise. If you are still awake by the time you get to your feet, start again!

A SIMPLE MINDFULNESS EXERCISE

Look out of a window and describe what you can see and hear, as if you are talking to someone who isn't there to experience it. Describe the details such as colours, textures, activity and sounds.

BREATHING EXERCISES

Box Breathing: Breathe in through your nose for the count of three. Hold your breath for the count of three. Breathe out through your mouth for the count of three. Hold the end of your breath for the count of three. Repeat the cycle three times.

Diaphragmatic Breathing: This type of breathing encourages us to inflate our lungs more efficiently and, if done properly, has a relaxing effect on the body. The best way to learn is to lie on your back on a bed or on the floor. Put a hand below your ribcage, above your belly button. Imagine there is a balloon under your hand. As you breathe out, push down, as if deflating the balloon. As you breathe in, your hand should rise up, as if the balloon is inflating. In reality, a deep breath into the bottom of your lungs pushes the diaphragm down which makes the abdomen rise up. It takes time to get used to this way of breathing. YouTube might be helpful. Once you feel confident in breathing this way, aim to do three diaphragmatic breaths four to five times a day. It will help you feel generally calmer and will prevent a build-up of tension in your chest and back.

Alternate Nostril Breathing: This breathing technique is often used in yoga. Press on your right nostril, to occlude it, and breathe in slowly through your left nostril. Release your right nostril. Press on your left nostril, to occlude it, breathe out through your right nostril then back in through your right nostril. Repeat three times.

Physiological Sigh: This is a technique which apparently helps to reduce the emotion in a highly charged situation, such as acute anxiety or anger. Breathe in through your nose, followed by a second quick breath in through your nose (to open up all the tiny airsacs in your lungs) then breathe slowly out through your mouth until your lungs feel completely empty. You will find demonstrations of this technique on YouTube.

USEFUL ADVICE FOR EYES

If you're spending a lot of time working at a screen, you might be interested in the 20:20:20 rule. Every 20 minutes, look at something 20 feet away for 20 seconds. (I suggest on the hour, twenty past the hour and twenty to the hour.)

The eye muscles contract to help us see things close up and relax when we look at things in the distance. Working at a screen for long periods puts a lot of strain on the eyes so this exercise is a useful way to look after your eyes.

NOTES

Printed in Great Britain
by Amazon